Type 2 Di

CW00351047

User's Manual on How to Treat Type 2 Diabetes using Natural Supplements.

Hillary A. Charles

Table of Contents

INTRODUCTION

Type 2 diabetes (T2D) is more prevalent than type 1 diabetes with about 90 to 95 percent of individuals with diabetes having Type 2 Diabetes (T2D). Based on the Centres for Disease Control and Prevention's statement, 30.3 million People in America, or 9.4% of the united states populace have diabetes.

There may be multiple reasons behind type II diabetes. A number of the reasons can be carrying excess fat, high blood circulation pressure, having an unhealthy diet, taking too much stress, hormone imbalance, certain medications and leading a sedentary lifestyle. Though type II diabetes can be reversed.

In this guide you will discover how you can attain your ideal body weight, improve your digestive health, gain energy, live an active life, and feel the best you've ever felt in years.

CHAPTER 1

Type II diabetes

Type II diabetes is more prevalent than Type I diabetes in India. Type II diabetes usually happens to folks who are above age 40. This sort of diabetes is triggered credited to insulin level of resistance. In cases like this, the pancreas produces insulin however the body struggles to react to it properly. There may be multiple reasons behind type II diabetes. A number of the reasons can be carrying excess fat, high blood circulation pressure, having an unhealthy diet, taking too much stress, hormone imbalance, certain medications and leading a sedentary lifestyle. Though type II diabetes can be reversed.

know some natural ways where you can treat diabetes at home:

What not to eat:

There are a few foods which can negatively impact your

diabetes. So, the very first thing you must do is to eliminate these food types from your daily diet.

1. Refined sugars - Everybody knows that glucose, until it is within its easiest form, is bad for individuals experiencing diabetes. When consumed, refined sugars spikes the bloodstream sugar quickly. Sometimes even the natural form like honey can result in an unexpected spike in the blood sugar. So, it's easier to avoid sophisticated sugar you should if you are a diabetic.

2. Wholegrains - Grains which have gluten in them should be prevented. Gluten is associated with diabetes as its intake can cause leaky gut resulting in inflammation which can result in auto immune system diseases.

3. Alcohol - Alcoholic beverages usage is straight related to diabetes. Alcoholic beverages not only problems your liver organ but also episodes the pancreas that produces insulin. Diabetes is associated with usage of heavy alcoholic beverages which is 2-3 glasses each day. Ale should especially be prevented as they have a great deal of carbohydrates.

4. Cow's milk - Exactly like wholegrains, cow milk can result in the disease fighting capability which can result in inflammation. Milk via sheep and goat is not dangerous in fact it can help to keep up the blood glucose level. However, the standard cow milk can be dangerous for you if you suffer from diabetes.

5. GMO foods - GMO foods are capable to market diabetes along with leading to liver organ and kidney diseases. Choose products that are called GMO-free.

What things to eat and do

Cinnamon

Cinnamon contains a bioactive substance that will help to battle and stop diabetes. Cinnamon may stimulate the insulin activity and therefore regulate the bloodstream sugars level. As more than anything is bad, similarly cinnamon if used excess can boost the risk of liver organ damage credited to a substance called coumarin within it. The real cinnamon, not the main one obtains shops (Cassia cinnamon) is safer to have.

How to consume cinnamon

- Blend half or one teaspoon of grounded cinnamon with tepid to warm water and also have it once daily.

- Boil natural cinnamon in 2 cups of water. Allow it cool for thirty minutes and also have it daily.

Aloe vera

Aloe vera is easily within Indian households. Though it's bitter in flavour, but combing it with buttermilk helps it be flavour better. Usually, aloe vera is utilized for beauty purposes but as they have anti-inflammatory properties it can heal the wounds. Because of its anti-inflammatory properties, it is stated to regulate the blood sugar.

Jamun

Jamun and its own leaves are actually helpful in decreasing the blood sugar. Consuming around 100 grams of Jamun every day is thought to show huge improvement in your blood sugar.

Vitamin C

Vitamin C isn't just good for pores and skin also for diabetes. Recent studies show that consuming around 600 mg of Supplement C daily can enhance the bloodstream glucose level significantly. Individuals who have persistent diabetes should consume foods abundant with Supplement C every day. Some foods abundant with Supplement C are amla, orange, tomato and blueberry.

Exercise

One of the primary reasons for type II diabetes has been overweight. Almost any physical activity, whether it is yoga exercise, Zumba, aerobics, gymming, playing sports activities can significantly improve bloodstream sugars level by keeping your weight. In addition, walking every day can help reduce the bloodstream sugar level greatly.

CHAPTER 2

Diabetes Herbs

The herbs and plant derivatives have been employed traditionally by indigenous people in the treating diabetes, in the areas where they grow.

Bauhinia forficata and Myrcia uniflorae

Bauhinia forficata grows in SOUTH USA, and can be used in Brazilian natural cures. This herb has been known as 'veggie insulin'. Myrcia uniflora is also broadly employed in SOUTH USA. Studies using the natural herbs as tea infusions claim that their hypoglycaemic results are overrated.

Coccinia indica

Coccinia indica is also called the 'ivy gourd' and grows wild over the Indian subcontinent. Typically used in ayurverdic remedies, the plant has been found to contain insulin-mimetic properties (i.electronic; it mimics the function of insulin).

Significant changes in glycaemic control have been reported in studies involving coccinia indica, and experts think that it ought to be studied further.

Ficus carica

Ficus carica, or fig-leaf, established fact as a diabetic treatment in Spain and South-western European countries, but its energetic component is unfamiliar. Some studies on pets claim that fig-leaf facilitates blood sugar uptake.

The efficacy of the plant is, however, still yet to be validated in the treating diabetes.

Ocimum sanctum

Ocimum sanctum can be an herb used in traditional ayurverdic practises, and is often known as holy basil. A managed clinical trial demonstrated a positive influence on postprandial and fasting sugar, and experts forecast that the natural herb could improve the working of beta cellular material, and facilitate the insulin secretion process.

Okra

Okra is gaining a reputation as a superfood for individuals at the chance of diabetes

Okra is fast gaining a reputation as a so-called 'superfood' for individuals with or vulnerable to diabetes or malignancy.

Commonly known as ladyfingers, or by its natural names Abelmoschus esculentus and Hibiscus esculentus, okra may have an optimistic influence on blood sugar control, among a great many other health benefits.

Opuntia streptacantha

Opuntia streptacantha (nopal) is often known as the prickly-pear cactus in the arid areas where it grows.

Inhabitants of the Mexican desert have traditionally employed the flower in glucose control. Intestinal glucose uptake may be suffering from some properties of the plant, and animal studies have found significant decreases in postprandial glucose and HbA1c.

Once more, to validate the prickly-pear cactus as a highly

effective method of aiding diabetics, long-term clinical tests are needed.

Further herbs which have been studied, and could have results for diabetics include:

- Berberine.

- Cinnamomym tamala.

- Curry.

- Eugenia jambolana.

- Gingko.

- Phyllanthus amarus.

- Pterocarpus marsupium.

- Solanum torvum and.

- Vinca rosea

CHAPTER 3

Herbs and supplements for type 2 diabetes

7 herbs and supplements

Listed below are seven herbs and supplements which may be of great benefit to people who have type 2 diabetes.

1. Aloe vera

Aloe vera is a common herb numerous different use. Many people know about its benefits for skincare, but it could likewise have other benefits, including slowing the improvement of type 2 diabetes.

One review, published in 2013, viewed the utilization of aloe vera to take care of symptoms of diabetes in rats. Results recommended that aloe vera will help protect and repair the beta cellular material in the pancreas that produce insulin. The experts believed this may be credited to aloe's antioxidant results.

The researchers needed more research into aloe and its own extracts to make sure of these results.

Means of taking aloe include:

- adding juiced pulp to a glass or two or smoothie.

- taking capsules which contain aloe as supplements

People shouldn't eat aloe vera skincare products.

Aloe vera juice may provide a number of health advantages.

2. Cinnamon

Cinnamon is a fragrant spice that originates from the bark of the tree. It really is a favorite ingredient in sweets, cooked goods, and other meals.

They have a flavor that can truly add sweetness with no additional sugar. It really is popular with people who have type 2 diabetes because of this alone, but it could also offer other benefits.

A 2010 review found evidence from studies involving humans that cinnamon may improve degrees of:

- glucose.

- insulin and insulin sensitivity.

- lipids, or fat, in the blood.

- antioxidant status.

- blood pressure.

- lean muscle mass.

- digestion

In another review posted in 2013, researchers figured cinnamon might trigger:

- lower fasting blood sugar levels.

- less total cholesterol and "bad" low-density lipoprotein (LDL) cholesterol.

- higher degrees of "good" high-density lipoprotein (HDL) cholesterol.

- a decrease in triglycerides, or body fat, in the blood.

- increased insulin sensitivity

It didn't may actually have a substantial effect on hemoglobin A1C. The A1C test is a typical test for diagnosing and monitoring diabetes.

Nevertheless, lipids, cholesterol, and insulin sensitivity are important markers for individuals with diabetes.

In both studies, the researchers remember that the results may rely on:

- the type of cinnamon, as the quantity of active component depends upon the type.

- the total amount or dose.

- the individual's response to cinnamon.

- other medications the individual may be taking

Most studies never have involved humans, so there's an insufficient evidence about how exactly cinnamon might affect people, including its likely side effects.

Researchers need to handle more research to verify the security and performance of cinnamon as a therapy.

People may take cinnamon:

- in a number of cooked meals and baked goods

- in teas

- as a supplement

Anyone who's thinking about using cinnamon supplements should talk with their doctor first.

3. Bitter melon

Momordica charantia, or bitter melon, is a medicinal fruit. Professionals of traditional Chinese language and Indian medication have used bitter melon for years and years. People can make the fruits and utilize it in many meals. Some researchers have been looking at its potential therapeutic uses.

There is certainly some evidence that bitter melon can help with the symptoms of diabetes. One review has mentioned that individuals have used many elements of the flower to help treat diabetes.

Research shows that taking bitter melon in the next forms can result in a decrease in blood sugar in a few people:

- seeds.

- combined vegetable pulp.

- Juice.

- supplements

Eating or taking in the bitter melon is definitely an acquired flavor, but taking supplements could make it more palatable.

There isn't enough evidence to aid using bitter melon rather than insulin or medication for diabetes.

However, it could help people rely less on those medications or lower their dosages.

4. Milk thistle

Folks have used milk thistle since old times for most different illnesses, and especially as a tonic for the liver organ.

Silymarin, the draw out from milk thistle that has received the most attention from researchers, is a substance with antioxidant and anti-inflammatory properties. They are the properties that could make milk thistle a good herb for individuals with diabetes.

Lots of the studies on silymarin are promising, however the research is not strong enough to recommend the plant or remove alone for diabetes treatment, according to one review published in 2016.

There look like no reports of significant side effects, and many people take milk thistle as a supplement. However, it is advisable to talk to a doctor first before using any supplements.

5. Fenugreek

Fenugreek is another seed that might help lower blood sugar.

The seed products contain materials and chemicals that help decelerate the digestion of carbs and sugar.

Additionally there is some proof that the seeds can help delay or avoid the onset of type 2 diabetes.

Findings of the 3-year analysis published in 2015 noted that individuals with prediabetes were less inclined to receive an analysis of type 2 diabetes while taking powdered fenugreek seed.

The researchers figured taking the seed resulted in:

- increased degrees of insulin in the torso, leading to.

- a decrease in blood sugar

lower cholesterol levels

The analysis involved 66 people who have diabetes who took 5 grams (g) of the seed preparation twice each day before meals, and 74 controls, who didn't take it.

An individual can:

- include fenugreek as a plant using dishes.

- add it to tepid to warm water.

- grind into a powder

- take it as a complement in capsule form

A variety of fenugreek pills is available here.

6. Gymnema

Gymnema sylvestre is a natural herb that originates from India. Its name means "glucose destroyer."

A 2013 review noted that individuals with both type 1 and type 2 diabetes who took gymnema showed indicators of improvement.

In people who have type 1 diabetes who took the leaf extract for one. Five years, fasting blood sugar fell significantly, weighed against an organization who received only insulin.

Other assessments using gymnema found that individuals with type 2 diabetes responded well to both leaf and its own extract over various periods.

Some individuals experienced:

- lower blood sugar.

- higher insulin levels

Using either the bottom leaf or leaf draw out may be beneficial. But once more, speak to your doctor about utilizing it before starting.

7. Ginger.

Ginger is another natural herb that individuals have used for a large number of years in traditional medication systems.

People often use ginger to help treat digestive and inflammatory issues.

However, in 2015, an assessment suggested that it could also help treat diabetes. The results demonstrated that ginger reduced blood sugar, but didn't lower bloodstream insulin levels.

As a result of this, they claim that ginger may reduce insulin level of resistance in the torso for type 2 diabetes.

However, the experts were uncertain concerning how ginger might do that, and they needed more research to verify these findings.

People may take ginger:

- with the addition of ginger powder or chopped, fresh ginger main to natural or prepared food

- brewed into tea

- as a product in capsule form

- by taking in it in a ginger ale

CHAPTER 4

The Best Herbs For Type 2 Diabetes

Although research is bound in this field, some herbs do show promise in treating type 2 diabetes, including:

- **Curcumin.** The chemical substance curcumin, which is situated in the spice turmeric, has been proven to both increase blood sugars control and assist in preventing the disease. Inside a nine-month research of 240 adults with pre-diabetes, those who required curcumin tablets (which can be found over-the-counter) completely prevented developing diabetes while a 6th of patients in the placebo group do.

- **Ginseng.** Ginseng has been used as a normal medicine for more than 2,000 years. Studies claim that both Asian and American ginseng can help lower bloodstream sugar in people who have diabetes. One research found that remove from the ginseng berry could normalize bloodstream glucose and improve insulin level of sensitivity in mice who have been bred to build up diabetes.

- **Fenugreek.** This supplement has been used as a medication so that as a spice for a large number of years in the center East. Great things about fenugreek for diabetes have been exhibited in both pet and human tests. In one research of 25 people who have type 2 diabetes, fenugreek was found to truly have a significant influence on controlling blood sugars.

- **Psyllium**. This vegetable fiber is situated in common mass laxatives and dietary fiber supplements. Psyllium in addition has been used historically to take care of diabetes. Studies also show that individuals with type 2 diabetes who take 10 grams of psyllium every day can enhance their blood glucose and lower bloodstream cholesterol.

- **Cinnamon.** Consuming about 50 % a teaspoon of cinnamon each day can lead to significant improvement in bloodstream sugars, cholesterol, and triglyceride levels in people who have type 2 diabetes.

- **Aloe vera.** This seed has been used for a large number of years because of its recovery properties. Some studies claim that the juice from the aloe vera place can help lower bloodstream sugar in people who have types 2 diabetes. The dried-out sap of the aloe vera herb has typically been found in Arabia to take care of diabetes.

- **Bitter melon.** That is a favorite ingredient of Asian cooking food and traditional Chinese language medicine. It really is believed to reduce thirst and exhaustion, that are possible symptoms of type 2 diabetes. Research shows that draw out of bitter melon can reduce bloodstream sugar.

- **Milk thistle.** This flowering plant is found round the Mediterranean Sea. It's been used because of its therapeutic properties for a large number of years. It really is sometimes known by the name of its energetic component, silybinin. Milk thistle may reduce insulin level of resistance in people who have type 2 diabetes who likewise have liver disease.

- **Holy basil.** This natural herb is commonly found in India as a normal medication for diabetes. Studies in pets claim that holy basil may boost the secretion of insulin. A managed trial of holy basil in people who have type 2 diabetes demonstrated a positive influence on fasting bloodstream glucose and on bloodstream sugar carrying out a meal.

CHAPTER 5

Herbal Products And Botanical Elements With Beneficial Results On Blood Sugar In Pre-Diabetes

Banaba (Lagerstroemia Speciosa)

It is commonly called as Queen's blossom (Physique one), satisfaction of India, large crape-myrtle or queen's crape-myrtle. It is one of the family Loosestrife. Queen's blossom is a deciduous exotic flowering tree growing up to 50 feet. tall, they have smooth curved, red-orange leaves having higher degrees of corosolic acidity. It decreases blood sugar (hypoglycemic impact), facilitates blood sugar transport into cellular material and reduces amount of triglycerides. Tea of the leaves is utilized against diabetes mellitus as well as for weight reduction. Banaba leaves have the ability to lower bloodstream sugar credited to acidity (triterpenoid glycoside) and other phytochemicals. The phytochemicals in the leaves of Banaba works at the molecular level by fine-tuning the broken insulin receptor, which is the reason for insulin resistance.

Banaba (Langerstroemia speciosa).

Glucose uptake-inducing activity of banaba extract was investigated in differentiated adipocytes utilizing a radioactive assay, and the power of banaba extract to induce differentiation in preadipocytes was examined by North and Traditional western blot analyses. Studies on the effectiveness and protection of banaba (Lagerstroemia speciosa L.) and corosolic acidity have been performed no adverse effects from it have been noticed or reported in pet studies or managed human clinical studies. The hypoglycemic ramifications of banaba have been related to both corosolic acidity as well as ellagitannins. Studies have been conducted in a variety of animal models, human being topics, and in vitro systems using drinking water soluble banaba leaf components, corosolic acidity, and ellagitannins. Corosolic acidity has been reported to diminish blood sugar within 60 min in individual subjects. Corosolic acidity also displays antihyperlipidemic and antioxidant activities.

Banaba also includes concentrations of soluble fiber and nutrients such as magnesium and zinc. It can help the body managing sugar and is really as such also effective in weight reduction and against weight problems. The hypoglycemic (bloodstream sugar decreasing) effect is comparable to that of insulin (which induces blood sugar transportation from the bloodstream into cells). The tea is restorative against problems such as diabetes, kidney and urinary problems.

Bitterwood (Quassia amara)

Commonly called as Surinam wood, amargo, bitterwood or quassia wood. Amargo is a little tree, 6 to 18 ft. tall. Amargo may control the bloodstream sugar possesses the phytochemical quassin. The results indicate that Quassia amara extract may be possibly valuable in the treating diabetes and associated dyslipidemia. This flower also possesses antileukemic, antitumorous, antibacterial and antifungal properties. It can be used in instances of anorexia nervosa, works well in chronic diseases of the liver organ and has anti-malaria activity. However, reproductive toxicity of Quassia amara remove in addition has been reported and its own action on sperm capaciation and acrosome response is recorded.

Silk cotton tree (Ceiba pentandra)

It is commonly called Kapok tree, silk cotton tree, sumauma or kankantri. It's very large majestic tree, with a conspicuously buttressed trunk. The kapok tree grows more than 200 ft. tall; with widely spreading branches. The silk cotton tree is cultivated for kapok. Oil from the seeds is utilized in edible products and the bottom seeds in animal feed. Ceiba pentandra has hypoglycemic effect and its own bark has been used as a diuretic, aphrodisiac, and also to treat headache, as well as type II diabetes. The results of experimental animal study indicated that Ceiba pentandra possesses antidiabetic activity; and therefore, is with the capacity of ameliorating hyperglycemia in streptozotocin-induced type-2 diabetic rats and is a potential source for isolation of new orally active agent(s) for anti-diabetic therapy.

Holy basil (Ocimum sanctum)

It is commonly called as Holy Basil, Tulsi, or Tulasi. Holy Basil is an exotic, much branched, annual plant, up to 18 ins tall, it develops into a minimal bush. Along using its spiritual significance, it also offers substantial medicinal indicating and can be used in Ayurvedic treatment. It could have an optimistic influence on fasting bloodstream glucose and on bloodstream sugar following foods. The herb is important in the management of immunological disorders such as allergic reactions and asthma. The juice of the leaves is utilized against diabetes and fever. It's anti-spasmodic properties, relieves stomach pains and assists with lowering the bloodstream sugars level.

Indian gooseberry (Eugenia jambolana)

They have common titles such as Java plum, jamun, jaman, dark plum. The Jamun can be an evergreen exotic tree 50 to 100 ft. high, with fragrant white plants and purplish-black oval edible berries. The juicy fruit-pulp consists of resin, gallic acidity and tannin. They have hypoglycemic (decreasing bloodstream glucose) and antioxidant properties. All elements of the java plum can be utilized medicinally and they have a long custom in alternative medication. The bark has anti-inflammatory activity and can be used In India for anemia, the bark and seed for diabetes which decrease the bloodstream sugars level quickly. In lab experiments, the dental administration of the draw out of jamun pulp raises serum insulin levels. These ingredients also inhibited insulins activity from liver organ and kidney. Studies on gastric mucosal unpleasant acid-pepsin secretion exhibited antidiabetic and antiulcer ramifications of remove of Eugenia jambolana seed in moderate diabetic rats.

Shatterstone (Phyllanthus niruri/amarus)

It really is commonly called as Child pick-a-back, gulf leaf flower, shatterstone, bahupatra or gale of blowing wind. Shatterstone is a common annual weed from the genus Phyllanthus which has more than 700 varieties. The plant matures to 1½ ft. high and has small yellowish flowers.

Physique 7 Shatter rock (Phyllanthus niruri).

The leaf and seed aqueous extract of Phyllanthus amarus

have been proven to enhances insulin resistance diabetes in experimental animal studies while an individual study on aqueous extract of Phyllanthus amarus has proven no influence on blood sugar in non-insulin reliant diabetics. The draw out of Phyllanthus niruri reduced blood sugar, suppressed postprandial rise in blood sugar following a blood sugar food, reduced hemoglobin glycation and increased complete and comparative weights as well as glycogen content of liver organ in diabetic rats. They may be anti-hepatotoxic (liver organ safeguarding), antibacterial and hypoglycemic. Other applications are against swelling of the appendix as well as for prostate problems. A fascinating aspect is the utilization of this vegetable for weight reduction (shedding pounds).

Ponkoranti (Salacia oblonga/Salacia reticulata)

It is often called Saptrangi or Ponkoranti. It really is a woody seed within the forests of Srilanka and India. The origins and stems of Salacia oblonga for diabetes treatment have been used thoroughly in Ayurveda and traditional Indian Medication for the procedure for diabetes.

Determine 8 Ponkoranti (Salacia oblonga).

It as a highly effective anti-diabetic and weight control agent. The body normally has alpha-glucosidase enzyme which break downs oligosaccharides into monosaccharides like glucose. The remove from S. oblonga binds to the enzyme and inhibits it. As a result of this inhibition, glucose is not released in to the blood stream. Within a double-blind Placebo-controlled, randomized trial, it was proven that Salacia reticulata boosts serum lipid information and glycemic control in patients with prediabetes and slight to moderate hyperlipidemia. This natural medication for diabetes treatment is well demonstrated and it is very successful in providing a remedy for the same.

Ivy gourd (Coccinia indica, Coccinia cordifolia or Coccinia grandis

It really is known by several brands; Calabacita, Calabaza Hiedra, Courge Écarlate, Kovai, Little Gourd, Tela Kucha, baby watermelon, little gourd, gentleman's feet or Tindola. Ivy gourd is an exotic place used as veggie and produced wildly throughout the Indian sub-continent. Ivy herb has been found in traditional medication as children treatment for various diseases. Ivy gourd can help regulate blood sugar and, subsequently, prevent or treat diabetes. Anti-inflammatory, antioxidant, antimutagenic, antidiabetic, antibacterial, antiprotozoal, antiulcer, hepatoprotective, expectorants, analgesic will be the reported pharmacological activities of ivy gourd. Components of the ivy gourd's root base, fruits, and leaves are thought to provide a range of health advantages. People take ivy gourd for diabetes, gonorrhea, and constipation. Its fruits are also used to take care of leprosy, fever, asthma, bronchitis and jaundice.

Aloe vera and Aloe barbadensis

Aloe, a favorite houseplant, has an extended background as a multipurpose folk treatment. The flower can be sectioned off into two basic products: dried out juice from the leaf and aloe gel. Latex from per cyclic cellular material obtained under the pores and skin of leaves may be evaporated to create a sticky material known as "medication aloes" or "aloe". This aloe juice provides the cathartic anthraquinone, barbaloin, a glucoside of aloe-emodin, and also other substances. Aloe gel is from the internal part of the leaves. It generally does not contain anthraquinones but will include a polysaccharide, glucomannan, which is comparable to guar gum. Aloe gel is utilized topically, but it has additionally been used orally for diabetes.

Although Aloe vera gel is way better known as a home treatment for small burns and other skin conditions, recent pet studies claim that Aloe vera gel can help people who have diabetes. A Japanese research evaluated the result of Aloe vera gel on bloodstream sugar. Experts isolated lots of energetic phytosterol substances from the gel which were found to lessen blood sugar and glycosylated hemoglobin levels.

Fenugreek (Trigonella foenum-graecum)

Fenugreek can be a plant found around India and its own seed products are usually used among the major constituents of Indian spices. Fenugreek, an associate of the legume family, has a bitter, maplelike flavor.

Fenugreek can be used to take care of numerous health issues, including insulin level of resistance, diabetes, poor hunger, irritation, digestive problems and menopausal symptoms. 4-hydroxyleucine, a book amino acidity from fenugreek seed products increases glucose activated insulin release. In pet experiments, it's been shown that dental administration of vegetable extract reduced the blood sugar levels. Administration of fenugreek seed products improved blood sugar metabolism and reduced hepatic and renal sugar-6-phosphatase and fructose−1, 6-biphosphatase activity.

Chemical substance constituents of the plant include saponins, a lot of that are glycosides of diosgenin. The seed products also support the alkaloids trigonelline, gentianine, and carpaine substances. Other the different parts of the seed products include several C-glycosides. The seed products contain up to 50% mucilaginous fibre. Other seed constituents include 4-hydroxyisoleucine, an amino acidity, and fenugreekine. Fenugreek is considered to hold off gastric emptying, sluggish carbs absorption, and inhibit blood sugar transport. It's been proven to increase erythrocyte insulin receptors and improve peripheral sugar utilization, thus displaying potential pancreatic as well as extrapancreatic results. Various the different parts of the seed products have differing activities. For instance, the element called fenugreekine, a steroidal sapogenin peptide ester, may have hypoglycaemic properties. Trigonelline, another element, may exert hypoglycaemic results in healthy patients without diabetes, but other studies show that fenugreek does not have any influence on fasting or postprandial blood sugar levels in non-diabetic subjects. You will find however studies which show that fenugreek may have part effects in babies of nursing moms who utilize this substance.

Since fenugreek is an associate of the Leguminosae family, which include peanuts, it is theoretically easy for someone with a peanut allergy to respond to fenugreek. However, this response hasn't been reported.

Garlic clove (Allium sativum)

It really is a bulbous perennial herb that matures to at least one 1.2 m (4 feet.) high. It produces hermaphrodite blossoms.

Allicin, a sulfur-containing substance is accountable for its pungent odor and it's been proven to have significant hypoglycaemic activity. This impact is regarded as credited to increased hepatic metabolism, increased insulin release from pancreatic beta cellular material and/or insulin sparing impact. Other studies including studies on aftereffect of garlic clove extract on blood sugar levels and lipid information in streptozotocin/alloxan-induced diabetic rats, alloxan diabetic rabbits have exhibited its antidiabetic activity. Aside from this, Allium sativum exhibits antimicrobial, anticancer and cardio protective activities also.

Cinnamon (Cinnamomum)

Cinnamon is a spice extracted from the internal bark of several trees and shrubs from the genus Cinnamomum. It really is often called dal chini, korunda, kurandu, kayu manis.Cinnamon increases blood sugar control in people who have type 2 diabetes. Probably the most energetic substance in cinnamon, known as methylhydroxy chalcone polymer; mimics insulin boosts blood sugar metabolism and effectively decreases blood sugar levels. Cinnamon also reduces serum triglycerides, LDL cholesterol, and total cholesterol.

Indian Kino (Pterocarpus marsupium)

Additionally, it is known as Vijayasar, Indian Kino, Malabar Kino, Benga, Bijiayasal, Piasal, Venkai. It is a deciduous moderate to large tree that can develop up to 30 meters high within India mainly in hilly region.

Pterostilbene, a constituent produced from wooden shows hypoglycemic activity because of existence of tannates in the draw out. Flavonoid portion from Pterocarpus marsupium has been proven to cause pancreatic beta cellular regranulation. Epicatechin, its energetic theory, has been found to be insulinogenic, improving insulin release and transformation of proinsulin to insulin in vitro.

Ginseng (Panax/Eleutherococcus)

Ginseng is a slow-growing perennial seed with fleshy origins, owned by the genus Panax of the family

Araliaceae. A number of products are called "ginseng." The mostly used are 3 different botanicals: Asian or Korean ginseng (Panax ginseng C.A. Meyer), American ginseng (Panax quinquefolius L.), or Russian or Siberian ginseng (Eleutherococcus senticosus Maximum). Reason behind Asian ginseng pays to in reducing the amount of sugar in the bloodstream. It has the capacity to improve the release of insulin from the pancreas and raise the quantity of insulin receptors. In medical studies, Asian ginseng has confirmed a primary blood-sugar lowering impact. American ginseng in addition has been proven to reduce postprandial glycemia in non-diabetic topics and topics with type 2 diabetes mellitus.

Previous study made to screen the result of syringin; a dynamic basic principle purified from the rhizome and main elements of Eleutherococcus senticosus, on the plasma sugar demonstrated reduction in plasma blood sugar in a dose-dependent manner one hour after intravenous shot of syringin into fasting wistar rats. The results claim that syringin comes with an ability to improve the discharge of acetylcholine from nerve terminals, which stimulate muscarinic M3 receptors in pancreatic cellular material and augment the insulin release to lead to plasma sugar reducing action.

Ginseng contains a family group of steroid-like substances called ginsenosides. Although there are numerous subtypes, ginsenosides are tetracyclic triterpenoid saponin glycosides considered to have various hormonal and central anxious system (CNS) results. Some ginseng substances show contradictory results; for example, ginsenoside Rg1 has hypertensive and CNS-stimulant results, whereas ginsenoside Rb1 has hypotensive and CNS depressant results. "Ginseng abuse symptoms" is a controversial undesirable impact that was reported in 14 of 133 long-term users of high daily dosages. These symptoms contain hypertension, nervousness, sleeplessness, epidermis eruptions, increased sex drive, and early morning diarrhea. The mostly reported side results include nervousness and excitation. Other results include headaches, hypertension, insomnia, estrogenic results including mastalgia, genital blood loss, and cerebral joint disease.

Blueberry (Vaccinium myrtillus)

It really is a low-growing shrub owned by the genus Vaccinium (family Ericaceae), bearing edible, almost black berries. These are carefully related to the Western bilberry. There are many types of blueberries can be found- including V. pallidum and V. corymbosum and develop throughout America. Its leaves will be the primary area of the place used medicinally. Blueberry is an all-natural method of managing or lowering blood sugar the leaves have a dynamic ingredient with an amazing ability to be rid your body of extreme glucose in the bloodstream. It really is a good astringent and helps alleviate swelling of the kidney, bladder and prostate.

Various impartial studies have concluded bilberry as a possibly effective use for treatment of eye problems associated with diabetes. Bilberry can help prevent diabetes related bloodstream vessel harm known Shape 14 Indian Kino (Pterocarpus marsupium). to affect the retina nerve and vessel functions. Anthocyanosides are bioflavonoids, chemical substance constituents in bilberry fruits regarded as responsible for a few of its vascular results. Anthocyanosides are believed to diminish vascular permeability and redistribute micro vascular blood circulation. They act like a few of the real estate agents in grape seed. The system in diabetes may be related to the high chromium content in bilberry leaf, but further research is required to determine this.

Collards

Collard greens will be the American British term for various looseleafed cultivars of Brassica oleracea. The vegetation is grown for his or her large, dark-coloured, edible leaves. These leaves offer high absorbable calcium mineral, iron, fibre, saturated in many essential nutritional vitamins like supplement C, supplement A, vitamin Electronic.

Collards are a good way to obtain niacin that really helps to reduce raised cholesterol and decrease the risk of getting diabetes. Much like most all veggie, collards employ a low glycemic index-slow release carbs no quick sugars spikes. Studies show that type 1 diabetics who consume high-fibre diets have lower blood sugar levels and type 2 diabetics may have improved bloodstream glucose, lipids and insulin levels. One glass of boiled collard greens provides about 8 grams of fibre. The Diet Guidelines for People in America suggests 21-25 g/day for ladies and 30-38 g/day for men.

Collard greens also contain an antioxidant known as alpha-lipoic acidity, which has been proven to lower sugar levels, increase insulin awareness and stop oxidative stress-induced changes in patients with diabetes. Studies on alpha-lipoic acidity also have shown lowers in peripheral neuropathy and/or autonomic neuropathy in diabetics.

Curry leaves (Murraya koenigii)

The curry tree (Murraya koenigii) is a tropical to sub-tropical tree in the family Rutaceae. Its leaves are found in many meals in India and neighboring countries. The leaves are usually called by the name "curry leaves" or "Nice Neem leaves" generally in most Indian languages.

Eating curry leaves twice per day has which can reduce blood sugar for nondiabetics and diabetics alike. That is a good natural herb to include within one's regular diet. Studies on antidiabetic activity of leaf components of Murraya koenigii on alloxan induced diabetic rats exposed it exerts hypoglycemic impact by increased insulin secretion and improvement of the glycogenesis process. The components were effective in regulating the biochemical indices associated with diabetes mellitus such as activities of glucokinase and blood sugar-6-phosphatase. Histological studies demonstrated that Murraya koenigii experienced protective results on damages triggered by alloxan to pancreas, spleen, liver organ and kidney, possibly by reducing oxidative stress and preservation of pancreatic cellular integrity.

Dandelion (Taraxacum officinale)

Often called dandelion, is a flowering herbaceous perennial plant of the family Asteraceae. As the dandelion is known as a weed, the herb has several therapeutic uses. Its leaves have been known diabetes avoidance herbs to lessen blood sugar. Utilize it in salads and green smoothies. Dandelion main stimulates the pancreas to make more insulin. Its main has a nutritional called inulin (not Insulin) that helps your body control bloodstream sugar. The chemical substance constituents include sesquiterpene lactones (bitters), taraxinic acidity (taraxacin), tetrahydroridentin B, triterpenoids and sterols: (taraxasterol, taraxerol, cycloartenol, betasitosterol) besides Supplement A, Supplement C, tannins, alkaloids, pectin, inulin, starch, potassium, beta carotene, caffeic acidity, and flavonoids (apigenin). It really is a good antidiabetic medication and can lower the blood sugar level. Assessments on diabetic mice show that dandelion remove can help regulate bloodstream sugars and keep cholesterol in balance.

Gumar (Gymnema sylvestre)

This plant's Hindi name means "sugar destroyer". It really is a native supplement of the exotic forests of southern and central India and Sri Lanka. Chewing its leaves suppresses the feeling of nice. This impact is related to the eponymous gymnemic acids. G. sylvestre has been found in silk medicine to avoid diabetes. They have herbal properties that help reduce and lower blood sugar. Even in type 1 diabetics, using Gymnema may also reduce insulin requirements. Gymnema gets rid of glucose from pancreas, restores pancreatic function. Studies have showed it exerts enzyme changes and sugar usage and has impact in controlling blood sugar level.

Prickly pear cactus (Opuntia dillenii)

Prickly pears are also called "tuna", "nopal" or nopales. Prickly pears are reddish fruits of common cactus that typically develop with flat, curved cladodes (also known as platyclades) that are equipped with two types of spines; large, easy, set spines and small, curly hair like prickles called glochids. It really is a traditional plant used as a folk treatment for high bloodstream sugar.

The very best hypoglycemic element of polysaccharides from Opuntia dillenii was dependant on preliminary testing and specifically studied for the antidiabetic ramifications of O. dillenii polysaccharide (ODP)-Ia in mice with streptozotocin (STZ)- induced diabetes. It had been suggested that ODP-Ia exerts its antihyperglycemic impact by safeguarding the liver organ from peroxidation harm and by keeping tissue function, therefore improving the level of sensitivity and response of focus on cellular material in diabetic mice to insulin.

Chamomile (Matricaria chamomilla) and chamomile tea

Chamomile or camomile is the normal name for a number of daisylike vegetation of the family Asteraceae. Chamomile tea shows some proof having the ability to lower bloodstream sugar and therefore prevent the development of type-2 diabetes and stop a few of the harm associated with high blood sugar. Studies have exhibited the consequences of chamomile warm water extract and its own major components on preventing hyperglycemia and the safety or improvement of diabetic problems in diabetes mellitus. Chamomile draw out demonstrated potent inhibition against aldose reductase (ALR2), and its own components, umbelliferon, esculetin, luteolin, and quercetin, have been proven to significantly inhibit the buildup of sorbitol in human being erythrocytes. These results obviously recommended that daily usage of chamomile tea with foods could donate to preventing the improvement of hyperglycemia and diabetic problems.

CHAPTER 6

10 Supplements to greatly help Lower Bloodstream Sugar

1. Cinnamon

Cinnamon supplements are either created from entire cinnamon natural powder or an extract. Many reports suggest it can help lower blood sugars and enhances diabetes control.

When people who have prediabetes - signifying a fasting bloodstream glucose of 100-125 mg/dl - took 250 mg of cinnamon extract before breakfast time and dinner for 90 days, they experienced an 8.4% reduction in fasting blood vessels sugar in comparison to those on the placebo.

In another three-month study, people who have type 2 diabetes who took either 120 or 360 mg of cinnamon extract before breakfast saw an 11% or 14% reduction in fasting blood sugar, respectively, in comparison to those on the placebo.

Additionally, their hemoglobin A1C - a three-month average of blood sugar - decreased by 0.67% or 0.92%, respectively. All individuals got the same diabetes medication during the research.

How it works: Cinnamon can help your body's cellular material better react to insulin. Subsequently, this allows sugars into the cellular material, lowering blood glucose.

Taking it: The suggested dose of cinnamon draw out is 250 mg twice each day before meals. For a normal (non-extract) cinnamon product, 500 mg two times per day may be best.

Precautions: The normal Cassia variety of cinnamon contains more coumarin, a substance that may damage your liver organ in high quantities. Ceylon cinnamon, on the other hands, is lower in coumarin.

2. American Ginseng

American ginseng, an astypement grown mainly in THE UNITED STATES, has been proven to diminish post-meal blood sugar by about 20% in healthy individuals and the ones with type 2 diabetes.

Additionally, when people who have type 2 diabetes took one gram of American ginseng 40 minutes before breakfast, lunch and dinner for just two months while maintaining their regular treatment, their fasting blood sugar decreased 10% in comparison to those on the placebo.

How it works: American ginseng may improve your cellular material' response to and boost your body's secretion of insulin.

Taking it: Take 1 gram up to two hours before every main meal - taking it sooner could cause your blood vessels sugar to drop too low. Daily dosages greater than 3 grams don't may actually offer additional benefits.

Safety measures: Ginseng can reduce the efficiency of warfarin, a bloodstream leaner, so avoid this mixture. It could also excite your immune system, that could hinder immunosuppressant drugs.

Harm to your gut bacteria's - such as from taking

antibiotics - is associated with an elevated threat of several diseases, including diabetes.

Probiotic supplements, that have beneficial bacteria or other microbes, offer numerous health advantages and could improve your body's handling of carbohydrates.

In an assessment of seven studies in people with type 2 diabetes, those who took probiotics for at least 8 weeks had a 16-mg/dl decrease in fasting blood sugar and a 0.53% decrease in A1C compared to those on a placebo.

Individuals who took probiotics containing several species of bacteria's had a much greater reduction in fasting blood sugar of 35 mg/dl.

How it works: Pet studies claim that probiotics may reduce blood sugars by reducing irritation and avoiding the damage of pancreatic cellular material that produce insulin. A number of other systems may be included as well.

Taking it: Get one of these probiotic with an increase of than one beneficial species, like a mixture of L. acidophilus, B. bifidum and L. rhamnosus. It's unfamiliar whether there's a perfect mixture of microbes for diabetes.

Safety measures: Probiotics are unlikely to cause damage, however in certain rare cases they may lead to serious infections in people who have significantly impaired defense systems.

4. Aloe Vera

Aloe vera also may help those trying to lessen their blood glucose. Supplements or juice created from the leaves of the cactus-like plant may help lower fasting bloodstream sugars and A1C in people who have prediabetes or type 2 diabetes.

In an assessment of 9 studies in people who have type 2 diabetes, supplementing with aloe for 4-14 weeks reduced fasting blood sugars by 46.6 mg/dl and A1C by 1.05%.

Individuals who had fasting bloodstream glucose above 200 mg/dl before taking aloe experienced even more powerful benefits.

How it works: Mouse studies indicate that aloe may activate insulin creation in pancreatic cellular material, but this hasn't been confirmed. Other mechanisms may be engaged.

Taking it: The very best dose and form are unknown. Common dosages examined in studies include 1,000 mg daily in pills or 2 tablespoons (30 ml) daily of aloe juice in break up dosages.

Safety measures: Aloe can connect to several medications, so consult with your doctor before utilizing it. It will never be studied with the center medication digoxin (15).

5. Berberine

Berberine isn't a particular herb, but instead a bitter-tasting substance extracted from the root base and stems of certain plant life, including goldenseal and phellodendron.

An assessment of 27 studies in people who have type 2 diabetes noticed that taking berberine in mixture with lifestyle changes reduced fasting bloodstream glucose by

15.5 mg/dl and A1C by 0.71% in comparison to lifestyle changes alone or a placebo.

The review also noted that berberine supplements taken alongside diabetes medication helped lower bloodstream sugars more than medication alone.

How it works: Berberine may improve insulin awareness and enhance glucose uptake from your bloodstream into the muscles, which helps lower bloodstream sugars.

Taking it: An average dose is 300-500 mg taken 2-3 times daily with main meals.

Safety measures: Berberine could cause digestive disruptions, such as constipation, diarrhea or gas, which might be improved with a lesser (300 mg) dosage. Berberine may connect to several medications, so consult with your doctor before taking this health supplement.

6. Vitamin D

Vitamin D insufficiency is known as a potential risk factor for type 2 diabetes.

In one research, 72% of individuals with type 2 diabetes

were lacking in vitamin D in the beginning of the research.

After 8 weeks of going for a 4,500-IU supplement of vitamin D daily, both fasting blood sugar and A1C improved. Actually, 48% of individuals got an A1C that demonstrated good blood sugars control, in comparison to only 32% prior to the research.

How it works: Vitamin D may enhance the function of pancreatic cellular material that produce insulin and boost your body's responsiveness to insulin.

Taking it: Ask your physician for a vitamin D blood vessel test to look for the best dose for you. The energetic form is D3, or cholecalciferol, so look because of this name on dietary supplement bottles.

Precautions: Supplement D may trigger mild to moderate reactions with various kinds medications, so ask your physician or pharmacist for guidance.

7. Gymnema

Gymnema sylvestre can be a natural herb used as a diabetes treatment in the Ayurvedic custom of India. The

Hindu name for the plant - gurmar - means "sugar destroyer".

In one research, people who have type 2 diabetes taking 400 mg of gymnema leaf extract daily for 18-20 weeks experienced a 29% reduction in fasting blood glucose. A1C reduced from 11.9% in the beginning of the research to 8.48%.

Further research shows that this herb can help lower fasting blood sugar and A1C in type 1 (insulin-dependent) diabetes and could reduce cravings for sweets by suppressing the sweet-taste sensation in the mouth area.

How it works: Gymnema sylvestre may reduce sugars absorption in your gut and promote cellular material' uptake of glucose from your bloodstream. Because of its effect on type 1 diabetes, it's suspected that Gymnema sylvestre may somehow help insulin-producing cellular material in your pancreas.

Taking it: The recommended dose is 200 mg of Gymnema sylvestre leaf remove twice each day with meals.

Safety measures: Gymnema sylvestre can boost the blood sugars ramifications of insulin, so utilize it only with a doctor's assistance invest the insulin injections. It could also affect bloodstream degrees of some drugs, and one case of liver organ harm has been reported.

8. Magnesium

Low blood degrees of magnesium have been seen in 25-38% of individuals with type 2 diabetes and are more prevalent in those who don't have their bloodstream sugars under good control.

Inside a systematic review, eight of 12 studies indicated that giving magnesium supplements for 6-24 weeks to healthy people or people that have type 2 diabetes or prediabetes helped reduce fasting blood sugar, in comparison to a placebo.

Furthermore, each 50-mg upsurge in magnesium intake produced a 3% reduction in fasting bloodstream glucose in those who entered the studies with low bloodstream magnesium levels.

How it works: Magnesium is involved with normal

insulin secretion and insulin action in your body's cells.

Taking it: Doses provided to people who have diabetes are usually 250-350 mg daily. Make sure to take magnesium with meals to boost absorption.

Safety measures: Avoid magnesium oxide, which can boost your threat of diarrhea. Magnesium supplements may connect to several medications, such as some diuretics and antibiotics, so consult with your doctor or pharmacist before taking it.

9. Alpha-Lipoic Acid

Alpha-lipoic acid solution, or ALA, is a vitamin-like chemical substance and powerful antioxidant stated in your liver organ and within some foods, such as spinach, broccoli and red meat.

When people who have type 2 diabetes took 300, 600, 900 or 1,200 mg of ALA together with their usual diabetes treatment for half a year, fasting blood glucose and A1C reduced more as the dosage increased.

How it works: ALA may improve insulin level of

sensitivity and your cellular material' uptake of sugars from your bloodstream, though it might take a couple of months to see these effects. It could also drive back oxidative damage triggered by high bloodstream glucose.

Taking it: Doses are usually 600-1,200 mg daily, used divided doses before meals.

Safety measures: ALA may hinder treatments for hyperthyroid or hypothyroid disease. Avoid large dosages of ALA if you have supplement B1 (thiamine) insufficiency or have a problem with alcoholism.

10. Chromium

Chromium deficiency minimizes your body's capability to use carbs - changed into glucose - for energy and increases your insulin needs.

In an assessment of 25 studies, chromium supplements reduced A1C by about 0.6% in people who have type 2 diabetes, and the common reduction in fasting blood sugars was around 21 mg/dl, in comparison to a placebo.

Handful of evidence shows that chromium also may help lower blood sugar in people who have type 1 diabetes.

How it works: Chromium may improve the ramifications of insulin or support the experience of pancreatic cellular material that produce insulin.

Taking it: An average dose is 200 mcg each day, but doses up to at least one 1,000 mcg each day have been examined in people who have diabetes and could become more effective. The chromium picolinate form is probable assimilated best.

Safety measures: Certain drugs - such as antacids as well as others prescribed for acid reflux - can reduce chromium absorption.

CHAPTER 7

6 Most severe Foods for Diabetics as well as for Preventing Diabetes

A number of the worst foods for diabetes - the foodstuffs that elevate bloodstream glucose, reduce insulin level of sensitivity and increase type 2 diabetes risk - will be the foods that are most common in the typical American diet.

1. Added Sugars

Diabetes is seen as an abnormally elevated blood sugar level. So, it's smart to avoid foods that cause dangerously high spikes in blood sugar. These are mainly enhanced foods such as sugar-sweetened drinks, devoid of dietary fibre that slows the absorption of blood sugar in the bloodstream.

Fruit drinks and sugary refined food items and sweets have similar results. These food types promote hyperglycaemia and insulin level of resistance. Plus, they promote the forming of advanced glycation end products

(Age groups) in the torso.

AGEs alter the standard, healthy function of cellular protein, stiffen the arteries, accelerate aging, and promote diabetes problems.

2. Refined Grains (White Grain and BLEACHED FLOUR Products)

Carbs like white grain, white pasta, and white breads are missing the dietary fiber from the initial grain. So, they increase blood sugar higher and faster than their intact, unrefined counterparts.

Inside a six-year research of 65,000 women, people that have diets saturated in refined carbohydrates from white bread, white grain, and pasta were 2.5 times as apt to be identified as having type 2 diabetes in comparison to those who ate lower-glycaemic-load foods, such as intact wholegrains and whole wheat grains bread.

An analysis of four potential studies on white grain consumption and diabetes discovered that each daily offering of white grain increased the chance of diabetes by 11%.

As well as the glucose-raising effects, prepared starchy foods also contain AGEs, which promote aging and diabetes complications.

3. Fried Foods

Potato chips, People from france fries, doughnuts, and other fried starches focus on a high-glycemic food, and then put on a wide array of low-nutrient calorie consumption by means of oil.

Plus, like other cooked starches, deep-fried foods contain Age range.

4. Trans Fat (Margarine, Shortening, JUNK FOOD, Prepared Baked Goods)

Diabetes accelerates coronary disease. Because the greater part of diabetics (more than 80%) pass away from coronary disease, any food that raises cardiovascular risk will be especially difficult for people that have diabetes.

Trans fat consumption is a solid diet risk factor for

cardiovascular disease; even a little amount of trans excess fat intake boosts risk.

In addition, with their cardiovascular results, saturated and trans fats reduce insulin sensitivity, resulting in elevated sugar and insulin levels, and higher threat of diabetes.

5. Red and Refined Meats

Initially, it may appear like the eating results on diabetes would be only highly relevant to carbohydrate-containing foods. The greater low-carbohydrate, high-protein foods in what you eat, the better; those foods don't straight raise blood sugar.

However, that is clearly a too simplistic view of the introduction of type 2 diabetes. Type 2 diabetes isn't only driven by raised sugar levels, but also by chronic swelling, oxidative stress, and modifications in circulating lipids (fat).

Many diabetics attended to think that if sugar and sophisticated grains and other high-glycaemic foods increase blood sugar and triglycerides, they ought to prevent them and eat even more pet protein to keep their blood sugar levels in balance.

However, several studies have finally verified that high intake of meats increases the threat of diabetes.

A meta-analysis of 12 studies figured high total meats intake increased type 2 diabetes risk 17% above low intake, high red meats intake increased risk 21%, and high refined meats intake increased risk 41%.

6. Whole Eggs

Eating 5 eggs/week or even more has been associated with an elevated threat of developing type 2 diabetes.

With regards to cardiovascular disease, eggs have been a controversial topic. However, for people that have diabetes, the study is not controversial; there are obvious links in many observational studies to large raises in risk.

Large potential studies like the Nurses' Health Research, MEDICAL RESEARCHERS Follow-up Research, and Physicians' Health Research reported that diabetics who eat even more than one egg/day dual their coronary disease or loss of life risk in comparison to diabetics that ate significantly less than one egg weekly.

Another research of diabetics reported that those eating one egg/day or even more had a fivefold upsurge in threat of death from coronary disease.

CHAPTER 8

15 effective herbs for diabetes

1. Gymnema Sylvestre

This plant generally is called 'sugar destroyer' in Hindi, and that means you can well imagine its diabetes-busting properties. The plant is packed with glycosides known as gymnemic acids. These essentially lessen your flavor bud's level of sensitivity to nice things, thereby decreasing sugar urges in prediabetics. Even those who find themselves already suffering from type 2 diabetes can control their sugars levels by using this plant. It does increase the enzyme activity in the cellular material, which leads to utlization of extra glucose in the torso. Additionally, it may positively impact insulin creation.

How To Consume Gymnema Sylvestre & The Dosage

You are able to consume it in the powdered form, make tea using its leaves or have pills. You may make tea by steeping the leaves in boiled drinking water for ten minutes. You can even add the natural powder to a glass of lukewarm drinking water and consume it. The dose is as comes after.

- Capsule: 100mg.

- Natural powder: ½-1 teaspoon.

- Leaves: 1 teaspoon

When To Take Gymnema Sylvestre

The optimum time to take Gymnema Sylvestre is each day or 20 minutes before meals.

Where To Buy Gymnema Sylvestre

You can purchase it online and at Ayurvedic stores or pharmacies.

2. Ginseng

Ginseng has been called an immunity boosting and disease-fighting natural herb for a long time, but experts have recently discovered that it also includes anti-diabetic properties. When you take ginseng, the absorption of carbs decreases, and the cellular material take up and use more blood sugar. After that, insulin creation in the pancreas also raises. All these give rise to a wholesome body that is less susceptible to diabetes. In the event that you currently have diabetes, this assist lower the blood sugar levels by 15 to 20%, much better than placebo, as shown by the study team from the University or college of Toronto.

How To Consume Ginseng & The Dosage

You could have ginseng root or powder. Chop the main and add it to boiled drinking water. Allow it steep for 5-6 minutes. You can even blend powdered ginseng in tepid to warm water and also have it. The dose is really as given below.

- Natural powder: 1 teaspoon

- Main: 2-3 g or 7-8 slices

When To Take Ginseng

Consume ginseng early each day and before dinner.

Where You Can Buy Ginseng

You can purchase it online or at Chinese medicine shops and Ayurvedic pharmacies.

3. Sage

Eating sage on a clear stomach can lessen the blood sugar levels significantly. It increases insulin secretion and activity, which really helps to suppress blood glucose in prediabetics and manage it in type 2 diabetics. After that, it also impacts liver function favorably, thus enhancing immunity. Although preferred as an addition to meats dishes, this supplement reaches its therapeutic best when it's consumed as tea.

How To Consume Sage & The Dosage

The ultimate way to consume sage is by means of tea. You can even include chew up sage leaves or add these to your meal or take sage supplements. To get ready sage tea, put boiling drinking water in a glass that contains 1-2 sage leaves. Allow it steep for five minutes. The medication dosage is as comes after.

- Leaves: 4-6 g/day

- Dried out leaves: ⅙-½ teaspoon

- Tea: 2-3 mugs/day

When To Take Sage

Consume sage tea or chew up sage leaves early each day on a clear stomach. You can sage leaves in your meal for lunch time and dinner.

Where You Can Buy Sage

You can purchase sage at food markets or online.

4. Bilberry

This is another effective herb for diabetes treatment which has shown immense medicinal potential. Not merely will it help type 2 diabetics, who have problems with high blood sugar, but additionally it is quite effective in dealing with diabetes mellitus. Bilberry consists of a substance called glucoquinine, which is chiefly accountable for reducing the blood sugar. Bilberry infusions can also help people whose eyesight has been jeopardized because of this disease. However, you ought to be careful if you are taking bilberry infusion along with diabetes medication as it can cause your bloodstream sugars to drop to dangerous levels. So, monitor your blood sugar regularly.

How To Consume Bilberry & The Dosage

Bilberry draw out is accessible and it is the safest way to regulate your blood sugar. Here's the dose.

Bilberry draw out: 10-100 mg with 25% anthocyanocides

When To Take Bilberry

You are able to consume the remove once each day and once at night one hour before dinner.

Where You Can Buy Bilberry

You can purchase bilberry draw out at a pharmacy, Ayurvedic stores, or online.

5. Oregano

Also called marjoram, this exotic herb of Spanish and Mediterranean origin may contain glycosides that lower the blood sugar in the torso. The water components of oregano show a glycosidase inhibitory activity in vitro.

The Rosmarinic acidity separated from the extract has been proven to boost the pancreatic amylase activity. In addition, it boosts the disease fighting capability. It can help in increasing insulin activity and mobilizes sugar in the cellular material, thus reducing the pace of carbohydrate development.

How To Consume Oregano & The Dosage

Oregano is regularly used in various cuisines. You should use fresh or dried out oregano in your meal, chew up the leaves, make oregano tea, consume diluted oregano essential oil or tablets. Make oregano tea with the addition of a teaspoon of dried out or fresh oregano to a glass of boiled drinking water. Allow it steep for five minutes. Scroll down for the medication dosage.

- Oregano capsule: 600 mg each day

- Oregano essential oil: 4-6 drops each day (diluted)

- Dried out oregano leaves: 1 teaspoon, twice each day

- Fresh oregano leaves: 4-5 leaves, twice per day

When To Take Oregano

It is advisable to drink oregano tea early each day. You can even chew up fresh leaves each day. Use dried out oregano for lunchtime and dinner.

Where You Can Buy Oregano

You can purchase oregano at any supermarket or online.

6. Aloe Vera

This fleshy leaf plant grows widely in India, South Africa, Mexico, Australia, and China. It's mostly used in aesthetic and pharmaceutical sectors. Aloe vera has been used for a long time to treat swelling, improve digestive function, prevent acne, and reduce hair loss. Recent scientific tests have discovered that aloe vera gel includes lipid-lowering and bloodstream sugar decreasing properties.

How To Consume Aloe Vera & The Dosage

Aloe vera juice and remove can be purchased in the market. You are able to consume them according to the instructions on the container. You can even prepare aloe vera juice at home. Have a 3-in . aloe vera leaf, draw out the gel and mix it. Add drinking water and lemon juice to dilute it. You can even consume aloe vera capsules. Here's the dosage.

- Aloe vera capsule: 300 mg each day

- Aloe vera juice or remove: according to instructions on the bottle

- Homemade aloe vera juice: 100 gm aloe vera gel

When To Take Aloe Vera

Consume aloe vera juice or extract early each day. You can have a capsule before lunch.

Where You Can Buy Aloe Vera

You can purchase aloe vera juice, draw out, or capsule at any Ayurvedic store or online.

7. Ginger

The mighty ginger is trusted in Asian cuisines and it is grown in China, India, Australia, Africa, and Jamaica. Like aloe vera, ginger has also been used in herbal medicines since ancient times. This aromatic spice can also help lower the blood glucose levels. Many scientific studies have confirmed that ginger helps to control the blood sugar levels by increasing insulin secretion and insulin sensitivity.

How To Consume Ginger & The Dosage

You are able to chew raw ginger, utilize it in your meal, drink ginger tea, consume ginger powder, use its essential oil, and add it among the elements in a cup of juice. Here's how much ginger you should consume each day.

- Ginger main: 1-2 inches

- Ginger essential oil: 3-4 drops

- Ginger in juice: 1 inch

- Ginger natural powder: ½-1 teaspoon

When To Take Ginger

Ginger tea is fantastic to start your entire day with. Stay away from eating ginger after 6 pm. Have a juice plus a little ginger juice before lunch time.

Where You Can Buy Ginger

You can purchase it at any supermarket or online.

8. Fenugreek

Fenugreek seed products and leaves are really beneficial to treat metabolic disorders and digestive problems. This herb is indigenous to Spain, India, Pakistan, Bangladesh, Turkey, France, Egypt, Argentina, and Morocco. It's been used since age groups to treat hair loss, pores and skin issues, and sluggish metabolism. This spice is also trusted in a variety of cuisines. A report verified that fenugreek seed products have bloodstream glucose-lowering results and may be used to treat type 2 diabetes.

How To Consume Fenugreek &The Dosage

The ultimate way to consume fenugreek is to soak the seeds overnight. You can even include the seed products and leaves in food arrangements. Here's how much fenugreek you should consume each day.

- Fenugreek seed products: 2 teaspoons

- Fenugreek natural powder: 1 teaspoon

- Fenugreek leaves: 200 g

When To Take Fenugreek

Drink fenugreek-soaked drinking water first thing each day. You could have fenugreek seed products or leaves during your meal.

Where You Can Buy Fenugreek

You can purchase fenugreek seeds and leaves at any supermarket or online.

9. Cinnamon

This strong-smelling spice, produced from the bark of cinnamon trees, is regularly found in South Asian cuisines and desserts. It really is an amazing natural product for diabetes and treat weight problems, muscle spasms, diarrhea, and common chilly. Many reports have verified that eating cinnamon regularly can help control high bloodstream sugar and therefore, it could be used alternatively medicine to take care of diabetes.

How To Consume Cinnamon & The Dosage

You will be able to consume cinnamon bark, natural powder, or pills. The dosage is really as stated below.

- Cinnamon stay: 2 inches

- Cinnamon natural powder: ½ teaspoon

- Cinnamon capsule: 500 mg each day

When To Take Cinnamon

You could have cinnamon tea each day and evening. Add cinnamon natural powder to your smoothie or juice for breakfast time. Have the capsule once in two times.

Where You Can Buy Cinnamon

You can purchase cinnamon at any supermarket or online.

10. Clove

Clove is a blossom bud that is popularly found in Indian, Pakistani, Bangladeshi, Sri Lankan, and Tanzanian cuisines. This aromatic spice has anti-inflammatory, antioxidant, and digestive properties. Research has verified that clove really helps to improve insulin awareness and decreases the degrees of bad cholesterol and triglycerides.

How To Consume & The Dosage

You can be able to consume clove by chewing it raw. You can even use entire or powdered cloves in food arrangements or consume clove tablets. Here's how many cloves you should consume.

- Clove: 2 for chewing, 5-6 in preparing food

- Clove natural powder: ½ teaspoon

- Clove capsule: 500 mg each day

When To Take

Soak 3-4 cloves in a glass of drinking water overnight and drink it each day. Use entire or powdered cloves in your meal for your meal. Take 2-3 clove pills in weekly before dinner.

Where You Can Buy

You can purchase clove atany supermarket and clove tablets at an Ayurvedic store or online.

11. Turmeric

Turmeric is often found in Indian, Bangladeshi, Pakistani, and Iranian cuisines. This ginger-like spice provides color and a definite taste to food. Turmeric is also an Ayurvedic medication that is utilized to take care of bacterial infections, wounds, epidermis issues, and digestive problems. Research has discovered that a phytochemical called curcumin is accountable for turmeric's yellowish color and therapeutic properties. Curcumin is also accountable for using a bloodstream glucose-lowering effect. Actually, one study verified that patients with type 2 diabetes could lower their blood sugar levels by eating turmeric.

How To Consume Turmeric & The Dosage

You are able to chew a little bit of raw turmeric, take pills, or consume it in the powder form. Here's how much turmeric you should consume each day.

- Raw turmeric main: ½ inch

- Turmeric root paste: 1-2 teaspoons

- Turmeric powder: 1-2 teaspoons

- Turmeric capsule: 500 mg, twice each day

When To Take Turmeric

You will be able to chew turmeric on a clear belly and use its paste or powder in cooking or smoothies/juices. Take the tablets before your meal.

Where You Can Buy Turmeric

You can purchase turmeric at any Indian or Pakistani supermarket or order it online.

12. Neem

Neem or Azadirachta indica is local to India. In addition, it grows in the neighboring countries like Bangladesh, Nepal, Sri Lanka, and Pakistan. Neem trees and shrubs have shiny to dark green leaves that have many therapeutic properties. Actually, its bark and fruits are also found in traditional medications. Ayurveda says that neem has antidiabetic, antifungal, antibacterial, antiviral, antioxidant, and anti-inflammatory properties. Several studies show it possesses bloodstream glucose-lowering properties. This confirms neem's antidiabetic property as stated in Ayurveda.

How To Consume Neem & The Dosage

You are able to chew thoroughly washed leaves of neem or take neem paste or neem pills. Here's how much neem you should consume.

- Neem leaves: 4-5

- Neem paste: 1 teaspoon

- Neem capsule: According to instructions on the bottle

When To Take Neem

You should consume neem paste diluted in one glass of water early each day. Nibbling neem leaves each day is also effective. Take neem supplements before breakfast time once a day.

Where You Can Buy Neem

You can purchase neem supplements/tablets online or at any Ayurvedic store. You can even buy neem leaves at the neighborhood market or Indian supermarkets.

13. Shilajit

Shilajit is situated in the Himalayas, Altai Mountains, Caucasus Mountains, and Gilgit-Baltistan Mountains. It really is a tar-like nutrient essential oil that oozes out of the mountains. Its color can range between light brownish to darkish. They have antioxidant properties and has been used to boost muscle power, decrease the risk of cardiovascular disease, slow down ageing, and increase fertility. It has additionally been discovered that Shilajit can help stabilize the blood sugar.

How To Consume Shilajit & The Dosage

You are able to consume good quality shilajit supplements with dairy, honey or sesame oil. This is actually the dosage.

- Shilajit capsule: 100-300 mg each day

When To Take Shilajit

You may be able to consume it each day and before lunch/dinner.

Where You Can Buy Shilajit

You can purchase Shilajit online or at any Ayurvedic store.

14. Chromium

With regards to lowering bloodstream glucose, chromium is among the best supplements. It has gained recognition as a health supplement. Chromium keeps your carb desires at bay, decreases bad cholesterol levels, mobilizes excess fat, and enhances insulin level of sensitivity.

How To Consume Chromium & The Dosage?

Chromium supplements, such as chromium picolinate, chromium polynicotinate, and chromium chloride, can be purchased in the market. This is actually the recommended dosage.

- 100-200 mcg, twice per day

- When To Take Chromium

- You can take chromium supplements before lunch and dinner.

Where You Can Buy Chromium

You can purchase the supplements at any pharmacy.

15. Alpha Lipoic Acid

Alpha Lipoic Acidity (ALA) can be an antioxidant mainly within potato, spinach, broccoli, liver organ, candida, and kidney. It really is usually used to take care of fatigue, memory reduction, kidney disease, liver organ disease, neuropathy, and Lyme disease. It's been discovered that alpha lipoic acidity supplements can help lower the blood sugar levels and therefore, it is a powerful supplement for dealing with diabetes type 2.

How To Consume Alpha Lipoic Acidity & The Dosage

ALA supplement pills are the easiest way to provide the body with a supplementary amount of ALA. Dose is as comes after.

- ALA capsule: 600 mg each day for three weeks

When TO TAKE

Before lunch.

Where You Can Buy

You can purchase it online or at any pharmacy.

Acknowledgments

The Glory of this book success goes to God Almighty and my beautiful Family, Fans, Readers & well-wishers, Customers and Friends for their endless support and encouragements.